2 B____ __

Intermittent Fasting
FOR BEGINNERS

+

Intermittent Fasting
FOR WOMEN OVER 60

This book is dedicated to all those who love themselves and aspire to unlock the boundless possibilities within their age and potential.

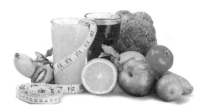

May the words in this book be a source of encouragement to pursue your goals, regardless of your age.

Emily William

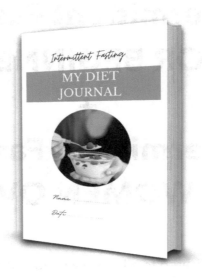

You can **download** and print your

Bonus: Diet Journal

using the link or by scanning the QR code
contained in the book.

BOOK 1

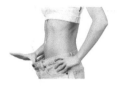

Discover the **benefits** of the Intermittent Fasting Diet.

Learn the **types** of intermittent fasting diet.

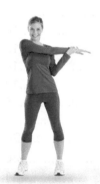

Choose the diet that best suits your needs.

Practice simple and impactful **exercises**, carefully illustrated and described.

BOOK 2

Follow **Your 28-day** Intermittent Fasting.

Discover many delicious **recipes**.

Follow **smart tips** and tricks to effortlessly reach your goals.

Find out how to **measure your physical** and **mental state.**

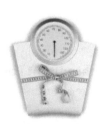

Monitor your well-being and **progress** with the appropriate tabs**.**

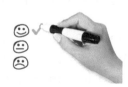

Table of Contents

Book 1

Intermittent Fasting for Beginners

Intermittent fasting has been getting a lot of attention lately, not just for its potential health benefits, but also for its historical and cultural significance. For countless generations, diverse societies have observed the act of fasting as a regular practice, often for religious or spiritual reasons. For example, during Ramadan, Muslims fast, while Christians do so during Lent. Greek philosopher and mathematician Pythagoras even recommended fasting as a way to improve health and longevity centuries ago.

Currently, scientists are investigating intermittent fasting as a possible way to handle a range of health problems, such as heart disease, diabetes, and obesity. This technique entails inducing the body into a state of ketosis during the fasting phase, causing it to use stored fat as a source of energy rather than glucose from food. As a result, it might help individuals lose weight, enhance their insulin sensitivity, and gain other health benefits.

How it Works

Intermittent fasting is a contemporary way of eating that requires switching between periods of eating and refraining from food. The concept is quite straightforward: while fasting, you are restricted from consuming any calorie-containing food or drink (with the exception of water, tea, or coffee). There are various intermittent fasting plans, such as the 16/8 plan, the 5:2 plan, and alternate day fasting, among others, which we will elaborate on in later chapters.

The reason why it is so popular is that it can help create a calorie deficit, which is often a key factor in weight loss. When you fast, your body eventually runs out of glucose and begins burning fat for energy instead. This process is called ketosis and can be very effective for shedding extra pounds, especially if you also exercise regularly and eat a healthy diet.

Body Changes After 60

As we get older, our bodies go through significant changes that can affect our overall health and wellness.

One of the most evident transformations that both females and males undergo are alterations in their hormones. The reduction of estrogen levels in women may lead to occurrences of sudden warmth, excessive perspiration during sleep, and changes in emotional state. Similarly, men can experience a decrease in testosterone levels, which can lead to fatigue, decreased muscle mass, and decreased bone density.

Another significant change that occurs with aging is the loss of muscle mass and strength. Engaging in regular activities and exercise can become tougher as a result, which can have a negative impact on overall physical functioning. As individuals age, their bones tend to become less dense, rendering them more susceptible to osteoporosis and fractures.

Metabolism also tends to slow down after age 60, making it more challenging to maintain a healthy weight. It can be quite vexing, however, it's crucial to bear in mind that these alterations are an inherent aspect of maturing and can differ from one individual to another.

As we get older, our immune system may become less effective in battling infections and diseases, thereby reducing its overall strength. However, staying active, eating a healthy diet, and taking care of yourself can help promote your overall health and wellness as you age.

Bear in mind that initiating the journey of nurturing your body and making healthy choices, which will yield long-term benefits, is within your reach at any moment!

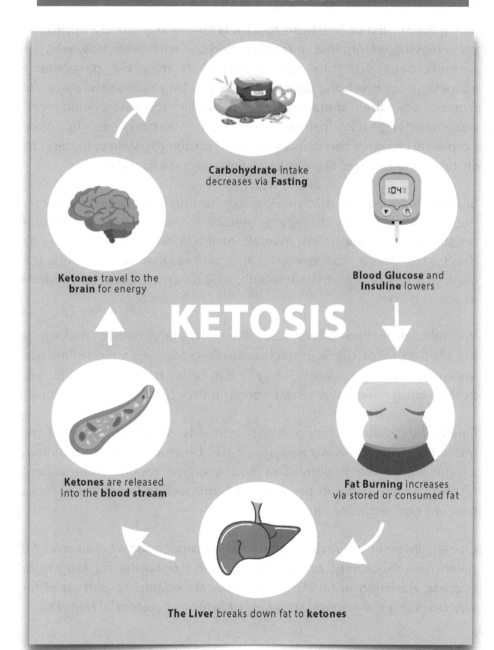

Carbohydrate intake decreases via Fasting

Blood Glucose and Insuline lowers

Ketones travel to the brain for energy

KETOSIS

Ketones are released into the blood stream

Fat Burning increases via stored or consumed fat

The Liver breaks down fat to ketones

Intermittent Fasting for Women over 60

Intermittent abstinence from food has become a trendy approach for achieving weight loss and enhancing overall health. However, for women over 60, this eating approach may be particularly advantageous given the unique challenges they face as they age. As women age, their metabolic rate naturally decreases, which can pose challenges in maintaining a desirable body weight. Also, hormonal changes can cause increased insulin resistance, leading to chronic health issues like cardiovascular disease and diabetes.

Studies have found that intermittent fasting can help counteract these challenges by boosting metabolic rates, reducing insulin resistance, and improving overall health indicators. The benefits don't stop there, as research also shows that it can enhance cognitive function and brain health, which can be especially critical as women age.

Intermittent fasting offers flexibility in dietary habits, making it possible to tailor the approach according to one's unique lifestyle and needs. Women over 60 may find it easier to adopt this lifestyle as they often have fewer social obligations or family responsibilities.

Finally, intermittent fasting is a sustainable long-term method for managing weight. As women age, it can be challenging to maintain weight despite a healthy diet and exercise routine. Intermittent fasting can be useful in breaking through weight loss plateaus and preventing weight regain.

Overall, intermittent fasting is an ideal approach for women over 60 given its adaptability, health benefits, and potential for long-term success. Assisting in tackling the obstacles related to getting older and boosting the general standard of living is a potential benefit.

Benefits of Intermittent Fasting

❖ **Lose weight:** Weight loss can be facilitated through intermittent fasting as it reduces your calorie intake while also boosting your metabolism.

❖ **Reduce inflammation:** By giving your digestive system a breakthrough intermittent fasting, it's possible to decrease inflammation levels in your body. This may potentially help lower the risk of developing chronic conditions like arthritis, heart disease, and cancer.

❖ **Improve heart health:** Intermittent abstinence from food has been found to be associated with positive indicators of cardiovascular well-being, including decreased levels of blood pressure and cholesterol.

❖ **Improve brain function:** According to some studies, periodically abstaining from food has been found to boost brain function and lower the chances of developing conditions that cause the brain to deteriorate, like Alzheimer's disease.

❖ **Reduce the risk of cancer:** According research, going without food for certain periods of time may have the potential to lower the chances of developing cancer. This may be attributed to its ability to reduce the accumulation of harmful substances within the body, thereby minimizing potential damage.

❖ **Increase longevity:** Intermittent fasting has been associated with living longer and having a lower chance of age-related illnesses.

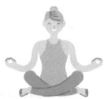

❖ **Improve immune function:** One potential benefit of intermittent fasting is enhancing the immune system by minimizing inflammation, and the production of white blood cells.

❖ **Reduce the risk of depression:** Research indicates that following a pattern of fasting intermittently could potentially decrease the likelihood of experiencing depression and enhance your overall emotional state.

❖ **Cut down the possibility of metabolic syndrome:** Current research suggests that implementing a schedule of intermittent fasting has the potential to decrease the chance of acquiring metabolic syndrome, a cluster of health conditions that increases the risk of diabetes and heart disease.

❖ **Improve insulin sensitivity:** Studies have found that adopting a fasting routine can enhance the body's ability to respond to insulin, potentially reducing the risk of developing type 2 diabetes.

❖ **Improve sleep:** There is a correlation between intermittent fasting and better sleep in terms of both quality and length.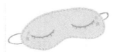

❖ **Improve gut health:** Refraining from eating for certain periods of time can enhance the well-being of the digestive system by stimulating the proliferation of beneficial microbes in the gut.

❖ **Increase energy:** By adopting intermittent fasting, you can enhance your energy levels by improving your body's ability to utilize insulin and boosting your metabolic rate.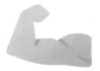

❖ **Cost-effective:** By taking periodic breaks from eating, intermittent fasting provides an affordable and accessible approach to enhance well-being and decrease the chances of long-term health conditions, which eliminates the requirement for pricey medication or therapies.

❖ **Improve skin health:** Adopting intermittent fasting as a regular practice may have a positive impact on skin health, as it can help to alleviate inflammation and encourage the process of cellular rejuvenation.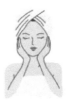

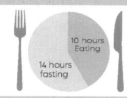

THE 14/10 METHOD
Good option for beginners

THE 16/8 METHOD
For fitness enthusiasts

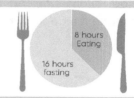

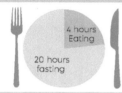

THE WARRIOR DIET
For the most experienced

Eat-Stop-Eat Plan
A long-term dietary habit

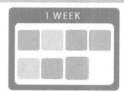

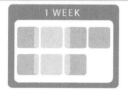

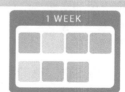

THE 36-hour METHOD
Not suitable for everyone

THE 5/2 APPROACH
Suitable for most people
(fewer calories for 2 days)

Types of Intermittent Fasting

There are several intermittent fasting techniques, each with a distinct pattern of fasting and eating. Let's take a look at some of the most common types of time-restricted eating.

The 14/10 Method

This method involves fasting for 14 hours and eating during a 10-hour window, making it a good option for beginners.

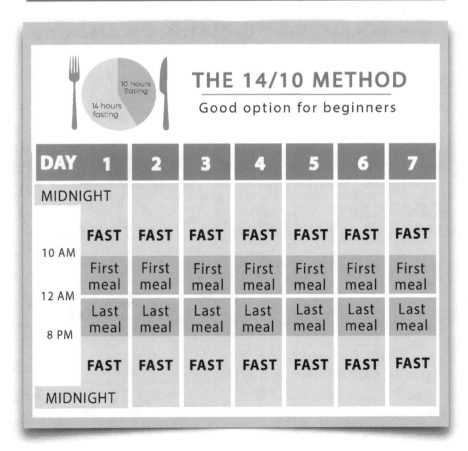

The 14/10 Method

THE 14/10 METHOD
Good option for beginners

10 hours Eating
14 hours fasting

DAY	1	2	3	4	5	6	7
MIDNIGHT							
10 AM	FAST	FAST	FAST	FAST	FAST	FAST	FAST
12 AM	First meal	First meal	First meal	First meal	First meal	First meal	First meal
8 PM	Last meal	Last meal	Last meal	Last meal	Last meal	Last meal	Last meal
MIDNIGHT	FAST	FAST	FAST	FAST	FAST	FAST	FAST

The 16/8 Method

The 16/8 approach to fasting requires refraining from eating for 16 hours, followed by eating within an 8-hour timeframe.

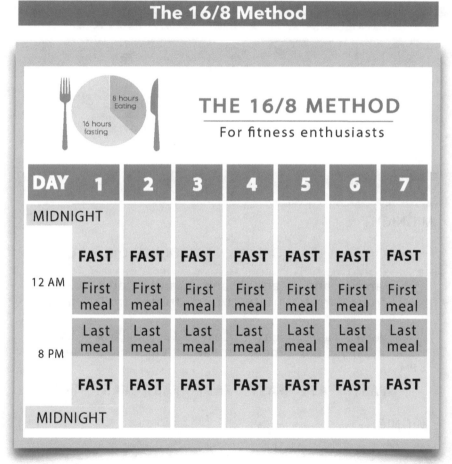

NOTE: This method is popular among fitness enthusiasts for its potential to improve body composition.

The Warrior Diet

The Warrior Diet, commonly referred to as the 20-hour method, requires fasting for 20 hours daily, with only a 4-hour window allocated for eating.

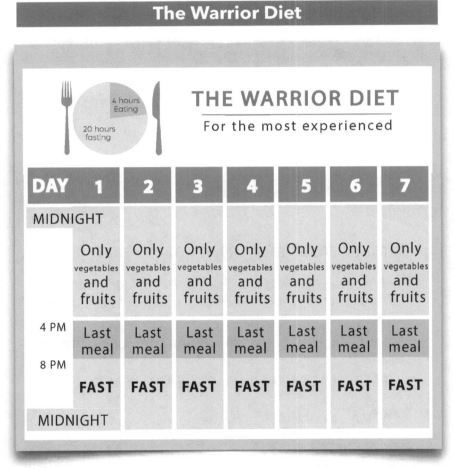

NOTE: This approach can prove to be difficult but highly beneficial.

The Eat-Stop-Eat Plan

The diet plan called Eat-Stop-Eat, also referred to as the 24-hour approach, involves abstaining from food for a whole day once or twice every week.

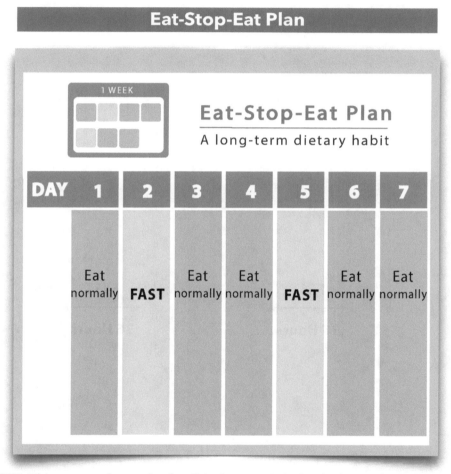

NOTE: This approach may be feasible for certain individuals as a long-term dietary habit.

The 36-hour Method

The 36-hour method, or ADF, involves fasting for 36 hours once or twice a week, but may not be suitable for everyone.

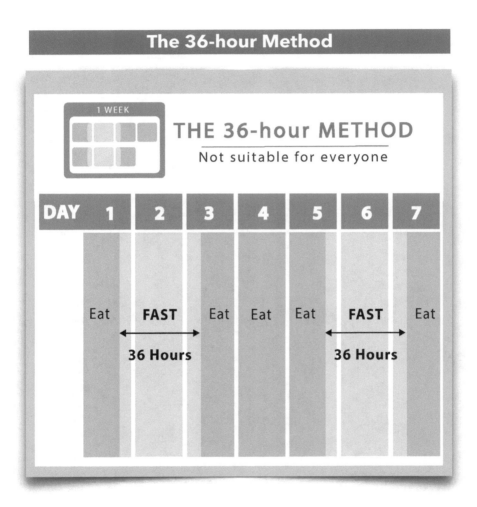

The 5/2 Method

Ultimately, the 5/2 approach consists of limiting caloric intake to 500-600 over two days that aren't consecutive, while maintaining a regular diet on the remaining five days.

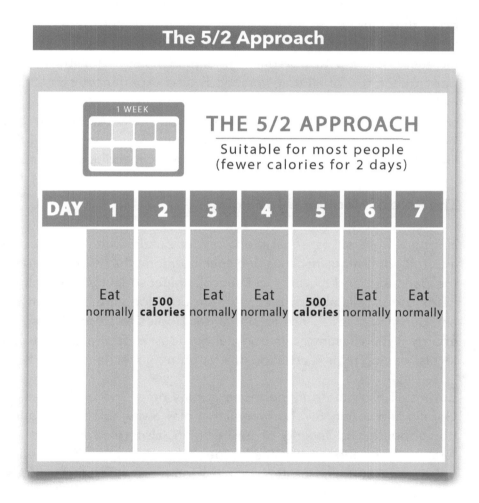

It's important to remember that intermittent fasting is not a one-size-fits-all approach and consulting a healthcare professional before starting any new regimen is important for safety and effectiveness.

The Body's Response to Fasting

When your body is in a fasted state, it goes through some changes to adjust to the absence of food. For instance, the level of insulin in your body goes down, which makes it possible for fat cells to release stored energy. This energy then gets used to power your body throughout the fasting period. Your physique undergoes a further transformation where the production of growth hormone increases, leading to potential benefits of muscle growth and fat burning. On top of all that, your body also experiences something called autophagy. This is a natural process that eliminates damaged or faulty proteins and organelles from your cells. Autophagy has been linked to several health advantages, including decreasing the likelihood of cancer and enhancing cognitive capabilities.

The Role of Hormones in Fasting

Hormones are an essential piece of the puzzle when it comes to intermittent fasting. Insulin is one such hormone that is produced by the pancreas, and it works to keep our glucose levels in check by helping our cells absorb glucose from our bloodstream. When we eat, our insulin levels rise to signal our bodies to store glucose as energy. When fasting, our body undergoes a decrease in insulin levels, leading to the activation of a fat-burning mechanism.

But insulin isn't the only hormone at play here. The body releases Ghrelin and Leptin, two hormones that play a vital role in regulating our appetite and feeling of full. Ghrelin, also referred to as the "craving hormone," stimulates hunger, whereas Leptin, the "feeling full hormone," helps us feel satiated for more extended periods. Intermittent fasting can help restore the balance of these hormones, which may lead to better overall health.

If you're planning to attempt intermittent fasting, keep in mind that it's more than just skipping meals or limiting your calorie intake.

The key is to provide your body with sufficient time to reset and regulate these vital hormones.

Through this approach, you may discover that you experience increased vitality, enhanced concentration, and an overall enhancement in your state of health.

Intermittent Fasting to Lose Weight

Intermittent fasting is a popular weight-loss strategy, which has found favor with older women over 60 because one of the key advantages of this approach is that it permits people to lower their calorie intake without imposing restrictions on the kinds of foods that they eat. This makes it a more sustainable weight loss approach, as it can be easier to stick with when you don't feel deprived or constantly hungry.

When a person practices intermittent fasting, they allow their body to go without food for longer periods of time. This leads to the body depending on its accumulated fat for fuel (the metabolic state referred to as ketosis). Instead of using glucose as fuel, the body starts burning fat, which ultimately leads to weight loss.

Beyond weight loss, there are other benefits to intermittent fasting that can support your weight loss journey. Intermittent fasting has demonstrated the potential to enhance insulin sensitivity, reduce inflammation, and boost metabolism. Nevertheless, it's crucial to keep in mind that unique factors such as age, gender, and initial weight could influence the effectiveness of intermittent fasting for weight loss.

Intermittent Fasting and Exercise

Intermittent fasting has become increasingly widespread to improve health and lose weight, which is well deserved, given its wide recognition and adoption. However, relying solely on fasting may not be enough to achieve your goals. That's where regular exercise comes in.

Exercise offers numerous benefits to support your weight loss goals, including preserving muscle mass, improving heart health, and boosting metabolism. That said, when exercising during intermittent fasting, you need to be mindful of a few things.

Firstly, pay attention to your body and adjust your workout routine accordingly. Intermittent fasting can affect your energy levels, so it may be necessary to opt for lower-intensity activities or modify your workouts, especially during the fasting period.

Secondly, when to exercise matters too. Some people prefer working out in the morning before breaking their fast, while others find it more effective to exercise during their eating window. It can be a process of trial and error to determine the most effective approach that suits your unique needs and fits into your daily routine.

For optimal advantages from working out, it's advisable to blend cardiovascular and resistance training exercises. Engaging in activities like running, cycling, or swimming can contribute to calorie burning and cardiovascular fitness, while weightlifting or body weight exercises can promote muscle growth and elevate metabolic rate.

Incorporating physical activity into your intermittent fasting plan has the potential to help you attain your weight loss and wellness objectives. However, it's essential to pay attention to your body's signals, modify your routine as required, and seek guidance from a medical expert before beginning any new workout program.

Your 7-Day Exercise Plan

When combined with a nutritious diet and consistent physical activity, intermittent fasting can prove to be a powerful approach to shedding pounds and achieving weight loss goals.

Here is a list of exercises that incorporate both cardio and strength training, along with instructions on how to perform each exercise, the recommended number of repetitions, and sets to get you started.

Keep in mind that the number of reps and sets may fluctuate depending on your fitness level and objectives. To prevent excessive strain on your body, start with fewer reps and sets and gradually enhance the difficulty as your physical fitness progresses.

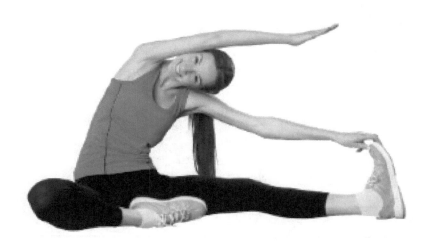

Jumping Jacks 1

Assume a sitting position with your feet and arms tightly together. Open your legs at the same time and raise your arms above your head. Repeat this action for 15 to 30 seconds, then take a 30-second break before repeating for a total of three sets.

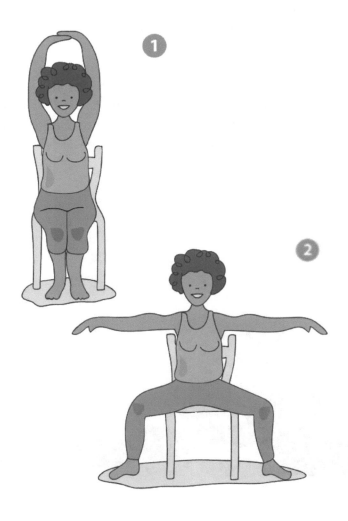

Jumping Jacks 2

Assume a standing position with your feet and arms tightly pressed together. Propel yourself upwards by simultaneously opening your legs wide and raising your arms up high over your head. When you touch down, ensure that your feet are spread apart at the same distance as your shoulders, and that your arms are resting by your sides. Repeat this action for 15 to 30 seconds, then take a 30-second break before repeating for a total of three sets

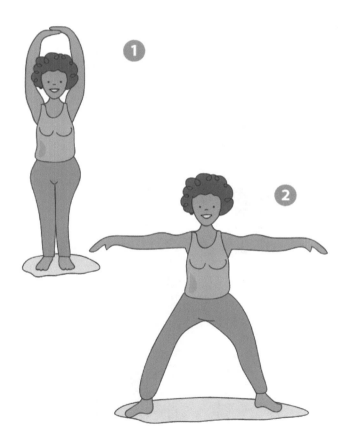

Squats

Position your feet at a distance equivalent to the width of your shoulders while pointing your toes slightly outward. Keep a straight back as you lower your body as if taking a seat on a chair. Descend as low as you can comfortably, then exert force on your heels to get back up to the initial position. Aim to perform 10 to 15 repetitions of this exercise for a total of three sets.

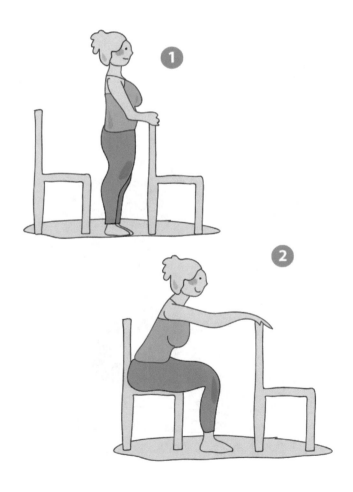

Lunges

Perform lunges by placing your feet apart at a distance equivalent to the width of your hips. Then, step forward with your right foot and gradually lower your body by flexing both knees at a 90-degree angle. Descend until your back knee is almost touching the ground. Lift yourself upward with your right heel until you reach the initial stance. Redo the process using your left foot. Perform 10 to 12 repetitions on each leg for three rounds.

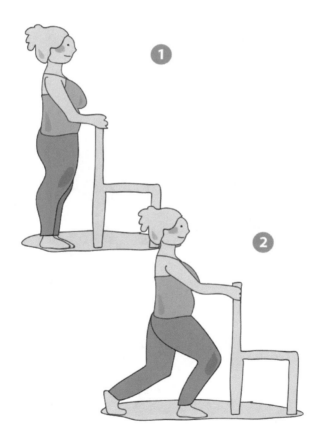

Wall Plank

Assume a push-up stance and gradually shift your weight to your forearms. Keep a straight posture from head to feet, and sustain the pose for roughly 30 seconds to a minute. Afterward, pause for half a minute, then redo the entire sequence three times.

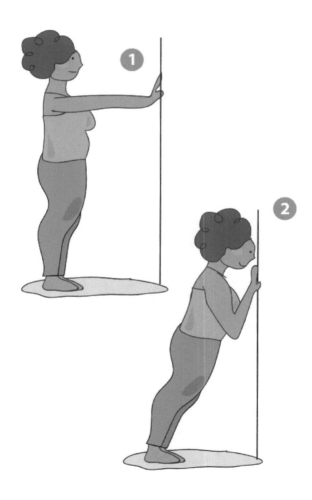

Biceps Curls

Adopt a sturdy stance by positioning your feet at the distance of your shoulders and take hold of a dumbbell in both of your hands. Keep your elbows near your torso and raise the dumbbells towards your shoulder area. Subsequently, bring down the weights to the starting point. Execute the exercise for 8 to 10 iterations and repeat the procedure three times during the entire workout.

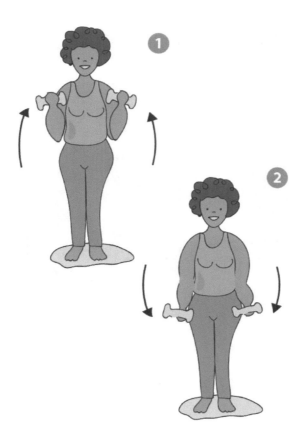

Wall Mountain Climbers

Assume the wall plank position by placing your hands at shoulder distance. Bring one of your knees towards your chest. Alternate knees for 30 seconds to 1 minute. Pause for 30 seconds and perform the workout again for a total of 3 rounds.

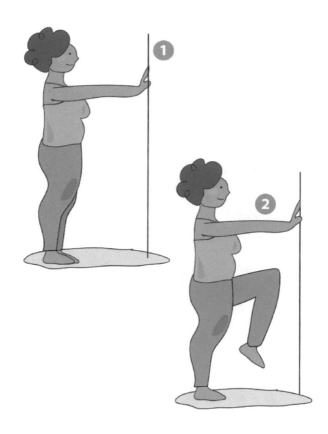

Intermittent Fasting and Meditation

Intermittent fasting and meditation are two practices that can complement each other nicely since they both have a positive impact on our overall well-being. When you fast intermittently, you may reduce inflammation, boost insulin sensitivity, and enhance cognitive function. Meanwhile, meditation can reduce stress and anxiety, improve mental clarity, and help you feel more at peace.

During the fasting period, meditation can be especially beneficial as it helps calm the mind and reduces feelings of hunger and cravings. Mindfulness meditation, for instance, can teach you to cultivate greater self-awareness and emotional regulation, which may come in handy when you're trying to follow an intermittent fasting schedule.

Moreover, combining intermittent fasting with a regular meditation practice may lead to a more mindful and purposeful approach to eating. This includes paying closer attention to the quality and quantity of food consumption during eating windows and being more attuned to your body's hunger and satiety cues. Incorporating meditation as a regular practice while intermittent fasting can yield immense advantages for both your physical and mental well-being. You should first seek the advice of a medical expert prior to embarking on any novel dietary or physical routine, such as intermittent fasting and mindfulness practices. Here are two examples of meditation practices:

Loving-Kindness Meditation

The process entails creating emotions of affection and goodwill directed towards both yourself, and individuals around you. Find a quiet place to sit comfortably and set a timer for a desired amount of time (e.g., 5-10 minutes to start).   Start by directing your concentration to your breathing. Afterward, silently iterate specific expressions to yourself, like

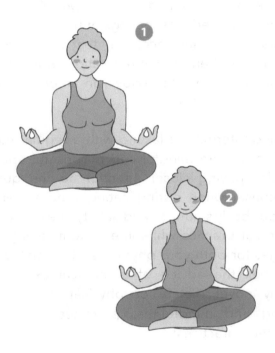

"May I experience joy, may I maintain good health, may I feel serene." After several minutes, expand this practice to include other people in your life, such as loved ones or even those you may be struggling with. With consistent implementation, this habit has the potential to foster increased kindness and understanding for yourself and those around you.

Mindfulness Meditation

To cultivate mindfulness and develop a deeper understanding of your thoughts and emotions without judgment, direct your focus to the present moment. Sit in a peaceful location and set a timer for your preferred length of time. Concentrate on your inhalation and exhalation as they flow through your body, allowing yourself to concentrate and be fully present in the moment. If your thoughts start to drift, gently redirect your focus back to your breathing. By regularly practicing this technique, it can promote self-awareness and improve emotional regulation skills.

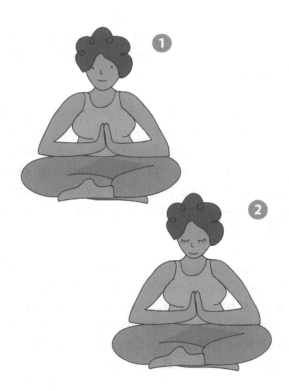

Dealing With Bad Days During Intermittent Fasting

"Starting Your Day with Purpose: Mindset Matters"

Starting your day with intention is an important aspect of managing your mindset when practicing intermittent fasting. Understandably, some days can be tough, and it's easy to fall into negative thought patterns when you're feeling hungry or fatigued. However, by setting a positive intention at the beginning of your day, you can help combat those negative thoughts and feelings.

An effective method to start your day with purpose is by inhaling deeply a couple of times. It may sound simple, but focusing on your breath and taking deep, slow inhales and exhales can help calm your mind and center your thoughts. Close your eyes, breathe deeply, and focus on the feeling of air filling your lungs and then leaving your body. One way to start your day off is by clearing your thoughts and with mental preparation.

After taking a few deep breaths, take a moment to set a positive intention for your day. Consider your desired achievements and create a mental image of yourself successfully attaining those goals. For example, if you have an important meeting or presentation, visualize yourself delivering a poised and victorious performance. If you're working on a project, visualize yourself making progress and feeling proud of your work.

It's crucial to concentrate on the emotions that will arise upon accomplishing your objectives. Consider the positive feeling of satisfaction and achievement that you will experience when successfully following through with your intermittent fasting plan for the day. Visualize that sensation and use it as inspiration to persist with achieving your objective. By focusing on the positive outcomes of your actions, you can be motivated to stay on track even when things get tough.

Based on my personal experience, I have found that setting a positive intention at the beginning of each day significantly helps in managing my mindset during tough times. When I'm feeling hungry or low on energy, I rely on reminding myself of my intention and visualize successfully achieving my goals. By doing so, I'm able to persist in maintaining my concentration and drive, even when confronted with tempting physical impulses that may otherwise urge me to quit.

"Prioritizing Your Health: Make It a Lifestyle"

When you're fasting intermittently, having a bad day can be tough. Giving utmost importance to your health and overall wellness should be considered imperative. There are a few healthy habits you can include in your routine to help you feel better when you're feeling down or overwhelmed.

Ensuring adequate water intake is another simple and effortless routine to incorporate. Hydration is crucial for upholding optimal well-being, and it can also enhance cognitive function and attentiveness. Drink 8 to 10 glasses of water every day and carry a water bottle with you to stay hydrated on the go. One effective strategy to enhance your mood and well-being while practicing intermittent fasting is to take a stroll. Physical activity has a beneficial impact on mental health, and a brisk walk can trigger the release of endorphins, thereby reducing stress levels. Furthermore, spending time outdoors and breathing in fresh air can refresh your mind and lift your spirits.

Mindful eating is a healthy habit that can make you feel better during your fasting period. Instead of snacking mindlessly or reaching for unhealthy foods, take the time to savor your meals and enjoy each bite. Be highly observant of the signals your body sends you when it comes to recognizing sensations of hunger or satiety.

When you start to feel full, it's best to stop eating as it can give you a sense of satisfaction and prevent you from overeating, which may result in unpleasant feelings of guilt and discomfort.

By integrating these beneficial practices into your everyday schedule, you can experience an improvement in your well-being and remain committed to achieving your intermittent fasting objectives. It's essential to find activities that you enjoy and that make you feel good, so don't be afraid to try new things until you find what works best for you.

For example, I find that drinking a cup of herbal tea during my fasting period helps me relax and feel more centered. Although the habit may appear uncomplicated, its impact on my general state of health and happiness is substantial. I also enjoy taking a yoga class or doing some light stretching in the morning to help me wake up and feel more energized for the day ahead.

Remember, dealing with bad days during intermittent fasting is all about finding healthy ways to cope and take care of yourself. You can enhance your mood, increase your overall energy, and improve your overall well-being by adopting healthy practices in your everyday life.

"Building a Support System: Surround Yourself With Positivity"

Dealing with bad days while intermittent fasting can be challenging, but there are several strategies you can use to make it easier. One of the most effective ways to stay on track is to surround yourself with people who share your commitment to a healthy lifestyle.

Finding a community of like-minded individuals can be a game changer when it comes to staying motivated and inspired. This can be especially helpful on those tough days when your willpower feels depleted, and the temptation to break your fast is strong. Being surrounded by individuals who can empathize with your struggles, provide assistance and motivation, can help you keep your progress towards your goals.

For example, let's say you're in the middle of a long fast, and you're feeling particularly irritable and short-tempered. You might be tempted to throw in the towel and indulge in some comfort food, but if you have a support system in place, they can remind you of your goals and offer words of encouragement to help you push through. Maybe your fasting buddy sends you a funny meme to lift your spirits, or your workout partner texts you some inspiring words to keep you going.

Being part of a community of like-minded individuals can also offer a sense of accountability. When you know that others are counting on you to stick to your fasting schedule, you're more likely to follow through. You might even find that you feel a sense of pride and accomplishment when you're able to resist the temptation to break your fast, knowing that you're not only doing it for yourself but for your fasting community as well.

Surrounding yourself with people who support and encourage your healthy lifestyle choices can be an effective way to stay motivated and inspired during intermittent fasting. Whether you join a local fitness group, or an online community, or simply enlist the help of a few close friends, having people in your corner can make all the difference on those tough days. So, reach out, and connect with others, and remember that you're not in this alone!

"Rethinking Rewards and Punishments: Treat Yourself Right"

Dealing with bad days during intermittent fasting can be tough, especially when you're feeling down and in need of comfort. But it's important to remember that turning to food as a reward or punishment may not be the best solution. Explore alternative methods of self-indulgence that don't include edibles.

You can opt for an alternate approach by submerging yourself in a soothing bathtub. This can help ease your mind and calm your body, which can be especially beneficial when you're feeling stressed or overwhelmed. One way to increase feeling relaxed is by including some drops of essential oils like chamomile or lavender.

Another way to treat yourself is to read a book. This can be a great distraction from negative thoughts and emotions and can transport you to another world for a little while. Whether you prefer a thrilling mystery or a heartwarming romance, choose a book that you know will make you feel good.

If you need a little retail therapy, consider buying yourself a new outfit. Whether it's a new shirt or a new pair of shoes, treating yourself to something new can give you a little boost of confidence and make you feel good about yourself.

I can recall a moment when I felt extremely low on a day of fasting, and my strongest desire was to indulge in unhealthy snacks and disregard the entire day. But instead, I decided to take a relaxing bath and read a book. I lit some candles, played some soft tunes and immersed my body into the warm water. Afterward, I curled up in bed with a good book and let myself get lost in the story. By the time I was finished, I felt much better and was able to resist the temptation of junk food.

Finding alternative ways to treat yourself during bad days while intermittent fasting is important. Whether it's taking a bath, reading a book, or buying yourself a new outfit, choose something that makes you feel happy and rewarded without relying on food. Taking small steps towards self-care can significantly impact your overall mood and help you overcome those difficult days.

"Challenging Negative Thoughts: Mind Over Matter"

It's important to remember that negative thoughts are not facts. They are just temporary emotions that can be managed with a bit of mindfulness and positive self-talk.

When negative thoughts arise, take a moment to acknowledge them and question their validity. Are they based on facts or fears? For example, you may have a thought like "I can't do this, I'm too hungry" during a particularly difficult fasting period. But is this true? Have you completed fasting periods before? Refresh your memory about the accomplishments you've achieved in the past and counter any negative thoughts that may arise with optimistic declarations and personal encouragement.

One effective technique is to replace negative thoughts with positive affirmations. Instead of expressing negative thoughts like "I'm incapable of doing this," switch to a more positive mindset by repeatedly telling yourself empowering affirmations such as "I have the strength and ability to overcome this challenge." By reciting these affirmations regularly throughout the day, you can help maintain a positive outlook and keep your mind focused on achieving your goals.

Another helpful technique is to practice mindfulness. Take a few deep breaths and bring your focus to the present moment. Observe the feelings in your physical being and the ideas in your cognitive processes without making any evaluations or criticisms towards them. By acknowledging your own negative thoughts, you can develop a heightened sense of self-awareness that may empower you to handle them more proficiently.

It's also important to believe in yourself and your ability to overcome challenges. Remember that bad days are a normal part of any journey and that you have the power to turn them around. You may find it helpful to write down your goals and reasons for intermittent fasting so that you can remind yourself of your motivation during difficult times.

In my experience, I have found that positive self-talk and affirmations have been incredibly effective in managing negative thoughts during intermittent fasting. There have been times when I've felt like giving up but reminding myself of my past successes and affirming my strength and resilience has helped me push through and stay committed to my goals.

"Focusing on Progress, Not Perfection: The Scale Is Not the Only Measure"

One thing to keep in mind is to avoid weighing yourself too often. While it's tempting to step on the scale every day to see if you've lost any weight, this can be discouraging on bad days when you don't see the progress you're hoping for. Instead, focus on other markers of progress, such as how your clothes fit or how you feel physically and mentally. This can help you see progress even if the number on the scale doesn't change as quickly as you'd like.

I recall an instance when I was feeling deeply unmotivated during my journey of intermittent fasting. Over the span of a few weeks, I had been adhering to my eating regimen. However, on this particular day, I sensed a strong inability to adhere to it. I was hungry, irritable, and just overall in a bad mood. When I stepped on the scale, the number hadn't budged, which just made me feel even worse. But then I remembered to focus on how my clothes fit, and I realized that my pants were starting to feel a bit looser. The minor triumph I experienced provided a boost in my morale regarding the headway I had made and served as an impetus for me to persevere.

Another consideration is to acknowledge and take pleasure in minor accomplishments. Even if you don't hit your fasting goals perfectly every day, it's important to acknowledge when you do make progress. Maybe you were able to fast for an extra hour, or you were able to resist the temptation to snack on something unhealthy. Recognizing these minor accomplishments can assist in maintaining your drive and generating progress towards your long-term objectives.

I remember another time when I was struggling to resist the temptation to snack on some chips. I had been doing well with my fasting up to that point, but for some reason, I just couldn't resist the salty crunch of the chips. But then I remembered that I had already gone several hours without eating anything, and that was progress in itself. I celebrated that small win and reminded myself that I could keep making progress even if I didn't stick to my plan perfectly.

Remember, intermittent fasting is a journey, and it's not about being perfect. It's about making progress towards your goals and focusing on that progress can help you get through the tough days. So, next time you're having a bad day, take a step back and focus on how far you've come, and the small wins you've already achieved. Celebrate those wins and keep moving forward. You've got this!

"Speaking to Yourself with Kindness: Be Your Cheerleader"

Sometimes it can feel like your body is fighting against you and every obstacle is getting in the way of your goals. It's crucial to keep in mind that it's acceptable to have rough days, and you're not the only one experiencing such emotions. One of the most effective ways to cope with these challenging times is by speaking to yourself with compassion and kindness.

When we have bad days, it's easy to get caught up in negative self-talk and beat ourselves up for not doing better. But this approach only makes things worse and can be demotivating. Imagine talking to a close friend who is facing a challenging situation and consider the words of comfort and encouragement you would offer them. Then, apply the same level of empathy and understanding to yourself.

For example, let's say you had a busy day at work and forgot to eat during your eating period, causing you to feel lightheaded and hungry. Rather than berating yourself for the mistake, try saying something like, "It's okay, I'm doing the best I can. I'm allowed to make mistakes, and I'll make sure to be more mindful tomorrow." By taking a gentle and understanding approach, you can help yourself feel more supported and motivated to continue with your intermittent fasting journey.

Personalized instances and stories can also bring this advice to life. For instance, perhaps you had a particularly challenging day where everything seemed to go wrong. You may have forgotten to pack your lunch, and the only food available at work was unhealthy junk food. Feeling frustrated and discouraged, you might start to doubt whether intermittent fasting is worth it.

However, by speaking to yourself with compassion and kindness, you can shift your mindset and stay on track.

In this scenario, you might say something like, "I know today was tough, but I'm proud of myself for sticking with my fasting schedule despite the challenges. Tomorrow is a new day, and I'll make sure to plan so I have healthy options available." By acknowledging the difficulty of the situation but also emphasizing your resilience and commitment, you can help yourself stay motivated and continue making progress towards your goals.

"Finding Joy in Life: Explore Your Passions"

One of the best ways to deal with bad days during intermittent fasting is to shift your focus away from food. Instead of focusing on what you are unable to consume, it may be beneficial to discover alternative ways of finding happiness and satisfaction. This could involve engaging in enjoyable activities such as spending quality time with family and friends, pursuing a personal interest, or contributing to your community through volunteer work.

For example, let's say you're having a particularly difficult day at work and you're feeling stressed out. Instead of reaching for a snack, take a few moments to step away from your desk and go for a walk. Taking a break and getting some fresh air can be a great way to clear your mind and refocus your energy.

If you're someone who enjoys being creative, try to find an activity that allows you to express yourself. Participating in artistic activities such as painting, writing, or playing music can provide a highly therapeutic and fulfilling experience.

Another great way to shift your focus away from food is to spend time with loved ones. Call a friend, spend time with your family, or even get a pet if that's an option for you. Spending time in the company of individuals or creatures that you hold dear can prove to be an effective means of elevating your spirits and fostering a deeper sense of belongingness to the environment that surrounds you.

Ultimately, engaging in volunteer work is an excellent means of experiencing a sense of personal satisfaction while simultaneously contributing to a beneficial change in the global community. Whether it's working at a local food bank or helping out at a community event, volunteering can be a great way to give back and feel like you're making a difference.

"Celebrate the Journey"

Sometimes, no matter how hard we try, we can't seem to stick to our fasting plan or may struggle with cravings and hunger pangs. However, it's important to remember that bad days are just a part of the journey, and it's essential to keep going and not give up.

To handle difficult days, a useful approach is to establish attainable objectives and recognize minor accomplishments during the process. This entails dividing your primary goal into smaller and more workable checkpoints that are simpler to accomplish. For example, if you're trying to lose weight through intermittent fasting, you could set a goal to lose one pound a week. Take time to acknowledge the minor accomplishments throughout your journey, like shedding a small amount of weight or successfully adhering to your fasting schedule for an entire day. These small wins may seem insignificant at first, but they can make a huge difference in your motivation and confidence.

In my own experience, initiating intermittent fasting posed a challenge as I struggled to resist the urge to eat for an extended period of time. Despite feeling discouraged, I opted not to quit and instead established realistic objectives. I started with a 12-hour fast and gradually increased my fasting window to 16 hours. Celebrating each milestone along the way, like making it through the first few hours of the fast, gave me the motivation I needed to keep going. Eventually, I was able to complete a 24-hour fast, which felt like a significant achievement.

It is crucial to take pride in the advancements you've accomplished, irrespective of their size. Make sure that you acknowledge your progress. Sometimes, we get so caught up in achieving the ultimate goal that we forget to acknowledge the progress we've already made. Pause for a moment and contemplate the extent of your progress from when you initially started to practice intermittent fasting. Maybe you've been able to stick to your fasting window for an entire week, or you've noticed that your clothes are fitting better. Whatever the accomplishment may be, be proud of yourself and use it as motivation to keep going.

"Visualizing Your Best Life: Belief in Yourself"

It's normal to feel frustrated or discouraged when you're struggling to stick to your eating schedule, especially if you're just starting. Although it may be challenging, there are strategies to triumph over pessimistic emotions and remain focused on achieving your objectives.

One of the most powerful tools you can use to stay motivated during intermittent fasting is visualization. Please pause for a moment and shut your eyes. Visualize the kind of life you aspire to have for yourself. Consider the individual you aspire to become and envision their appearance in your imagination.

Perhaps you envision yourself having increased vitality, enhanced mental clarity, and a stronger physique. Maybe you imagine yourself fitting into your favorite clothes or feeling confident in social situations. Keep your aspirations alive and trust in your capability to accomplish them, regardless of any obstacles.

Personalizing this technique can help you stay connected to your vision. For example, if your goal is to have more energy, you might visualize yourself going for a run or playing with your kids with boundless energy. If your goal is to fit into your favorite clothes, you might imagine yourself shopping for new clothes that fit perfectly or receiving compliments on how great you look.

It's important to have faith in your own potential for positive transformations to happen. Remind yourself of your past successes and the challenges you've overcome. Maybe you've lost weight before, quit smoking, or accomplished a challenging goal. Recalling those instances can enhance your self-assurance and serve as a reminder that you have what it takes to move forward.

"Taking Responsibility for Your Choices: Control What You Can"

You might find yourself feeling extra hungry, experiencing low energy levels, or just generally feeling off. Bear in mind that you hold the power to regulate your conduct and responses.

One thing you can do is to avoid blaming external factors for setbacks, and instead, take responsibility for your choices. It's easy to blame your mood or circumstances for your lack of willpower, but ultimately, it's up to you to decide whether to stick with your intermittent fasting plan or not.

For example, let's say you had a tough day at work and you feel like you deserve to treat yourself to a large meal. Resist the urge to indulge and instead, inhale deeply while recalling your objectives. Think about why you started intermittent fasting in the first place and how good you feel when you stick to your plan. Bear in mind that the ability to bring about favorable transformations in your life lies within you, and every day presents a chance for you to move closer to a more nourishing and happy version of yourself.

Remember that encountering obstacles is a normal occurrence in any endeavor. Everyone experiences setbacks and it's acceptable to have occasional slip-ups. The crucial point is to prevent these obstacles from defining your identity or impeding your progress. Direct your attention towards making progress and returning to the right path. Experiencing a single unpleasant day doesn't equate to personal failure, rather it's a natural aspect of being human.

For example, if you accidentally break your fast early, don't beat yourself up over it. Instead of viewing it as a failure, take the experience as a learning curve and determine how to modify your actions in the future to prevent repeating the same error. Maybe you need to plan your meals better or find a new way to manage stress.

"Coping With Stress: Find What Works for You"

One of the best ways to deal with a bad day during intermittent fasting is to find activities that help you manage stress and negative emotions. For instance, if you're feeling anxious or down, talking to a friend or loved one can be incredibly helpful. Sometimes just venting out your frustrations or talking through your worries can lighten your mood and help you feel more relaxed.

Another effective way to manage negative emotions is through yoga. Yoga involves physical activity coupled with breathing exercises and meditation, aimed at inducing a state of calmness and minimizing anxiety levels. Consistently engaging in yoga can promote a sense of calmness and equilibrium within oneself, especially when encountering challenging circumstances. A study conducted by the University of Michigan found that practicing yoga for just 20 minutes a day can significantly reduce stress and anxiety.

Participating in artistic expression can be a highly effective method of coping with stress and unfavorable emotions. Regardless of whether you choose to paint, sketch, or write, engaging in a creative endeavor can help you relax and allow you to communicate your emotions in a positive manner. This can be a great way to release any pent-up emotions and clear your mind, making it easier to stay on track with your intermittent fasting goals.

I find that going for a long walk or run outside can be incredibly therapeutic when I'm having a bad day. The fresh air and exercise help me clear my mind and release any tension I might be holding onto. I also make sure to listen to my favorite music or podcast while I'm out, which helps me stay distracted from any negative thoughts.

"Creating a Positive Environment: Clear the Clutter"

One effective way to cope with bad days while intermittent fasting is to eliminate clutter and distractions from your environment. While it may appear insignificant, taking a small action could significantly impact your emotional state and improve your concentration. If your environment is full of mess and diversions, it may lead to a feeling of disorder and stress, causing unwanted feelings and hindering your advancement.

So, start by decluttering your living space. This doesn't have to be a major overhaul; even just tidying up a little can help. Clear away any unnecessary items, organize your space, and create a sense of order. By cultivating a calmer state of mind and improving your concentration, you can experience enhanced emotional well-being and better adhere to your fasting regimen.

One approach to minimizing disruptions is to stop following social media that don't match your objectives. While social media can serve as a potent source of inspiration and encouragement, it can also be a cause of pessimism and diversion. If you find yourself feeling discouraged or triggered by certain accounts, it's time to unfollow them. Instead, follow accounts that align with your goals and promote a healthy lifestyle. Various types of profiles are posting, such as those that disseminate nutritious meal ideas, fitness guidance, and inspiring content.

Besides decluttering and eliminating distractions, surround yourself with positive images, affirmations, and whatever inspires you. This can include things like motivational posters, uplifting quotes, or photos of people who have achieved the goals you aspire to. When you surround yourself with positive images and affirmations, it can help you stay focused and motivated, even on bad days.

For example, if you're trying to lose weight through intermittent fasting, you might create a vision board with images of healthy foods, workout gear, and people who have achieved their weight loss goals. You could also write out affirmations that remind you of your why, such as "I am strong, and I am capable of achieving my goals."

"Solving Problems Rather Than Dwelling on Them: Focus on Solutions"

When you're having a bad day during intermittent fasting, the first step is to identify the problem. Is it hunger pangs? Feeling tired or low on energy? Have a headache? Perhaps you unintentionally disrupted your period of fasting by eating something that you shouldn't have?

After pinpointing the problem, the next step is to generate a range of potential resolutions through intensive brainstorming. For example, if you're feeling hungry, try drinking water, black coffee, or herbal tea to help suppress your appetite. You could also adjust your fasting schedule to allow for a longer eating window or try adding more fiber-rich foods to your meals to keep you feeling full longer.

If you accidentally break your fast, don't beat yourself up about it. Act promptly to realign with your fasting routine. Remember, intermittent fasting is a flexible approach, so you can always adjust your schedule to accommodate unexpected events.

Seeking advice from others can also help find solutions to your bad day during intermittent fasting. Consider contacting your community of individuals who are also practicing fasting or a close friend whom you trust, for necessary support and motivation. They could potentially offer you helpful tips or a different perspective that can assist you in overcoming any challenges you may encounter during your fasting journey.

In my experience, there have been days when I've struggled with intermittent fasting, especially during the initial phase. However, instead of giving up, I focused on finding solutions. For example, I found that adding more protein and healthy fats to my meals helped me feel full and satisfied longer, making it easier to stick to my fasting schedule.

"Expressing Gratitude: Appreciate What You Have"

Expressing gratitude involves recognizing and valuing the positive aspects of your existence. It's a powerful tool that can help shift your mindset from negativity to positivity, even on your worst days. When you shift your attention to the good things in your life, you can create a feeling of abundance and satisfaction, which can keep you inspired and dedicated to your intermittent fasting pursuit.

One method to foster a sense of gratitude is to spend some time each day pondering on the things that you appreciate. These can be diverse, ranging from a close friend or relative who is always there for you, a pastime or career that fulfills you, a mesmerizing sunset, or even the fundamental life necessities such as a safe home and food in the fridge. By dedicating moments to acknowledge the positive aspects of your life, you can counteract the negative feelings and emotions that often come with challenging days.

In my experience, expressing appreciation can be particularly beneficial in moments of stress or feeling burdened. For example, when I was in college, I often struggled with balancing my homework, job, and social life. On tougher days, I would take a few minutes to write down three things that I was grateful for, such as a supportive roommate, a good grade on a recent assignment, or a fun night out with friends. This straightforward habit enabled me to alter my perspective from a state of tension and unease to one of appreciation and optimism.

An alternative method for fostering gratitude involves keeping a journal where you regularly jot things you are thankful for. This can be a paper notebook or a digital document where you write down the things that you're grateful for each day. This can be particularly beneficial if you struggle to remember to actively engage in gratitude on a daily basis. By consistently practicing the habit of jotting down things that evoke feelings of gratitude within you, you can train your mind to focus on the positive aspects of your existence.

Assessing Eating Habits

Before starting, it's essential to assess your current eating habits to make sure you practice intermittent fasting safely and effectively.

When I learned about intermittent fasting, my curiosity was piqued, but I also felt a twinge of apprehension. As an individual who faced weight struggles, the idea of skipping meals brought about feelings of discomfort within me. But I decided to give it a try and started by keeping a food diary for a few days. I gained a new perspective on my eating habits after I observed how frequently I ate food. It became apparent to me that I frequently indulged in snacks when feeling unoccupied or stressed, and I had a habit of eating during late hours.

Using this information, I chose a fasting plan that worked best for me. Initially, I began implementing a fasting period of 12 hours from the time I finished dinner to when I had breakfast. Over time, I gradually extended this fasting window to 16 hours. Initially, it posed a challenge, but eventually, I discovered that my consumption of abundant water and herbal tea proved to be effective in providing me with a sensation of fullness and contentment.

Another important aspect of assessing your eating habits is looking at the nutritional value of your meals. It's crucial to maintain a well-rounded eating plan that includes a diverse array of fruits, vegetables, whole grains, and lean sources of protein. I realized that I was eating a lot of processed foods and not enough fresh produce, so I started making simple changes like adding more salads and swapping out sugary snacks for fruit.

Take note of any medical condition or medication that may impact your ability to fast safely. Suppose you have diabetes; in that case, you might have to modify the amount of insulin you take while fasting. In case you are unsure whether intermittent fasting is a suitable choice for you or have any concerns, it is advisable to seek the guidance of a healthcare professional.

Assessing your eating habits is not only important for successful intermittent fasting but also for your overall health and wellness. By identifying patterns and making necessary changes, you can improve your relationship with food and feel better both physically and mentally.

Setting Realistic Goals

Setting realistic goals is a crucial step to take before starting intermittent fasting. One way to remain encouraged and committed to your fasting regimen is to persevere diligently and stay focused on your goals. Your primary goal could be weight loss or improved health, and it's essential to establish smaller, achievable goals to work towards.

For instance, suppose your primary goal is weight loss. In this scenario, you could establish a target of shedding 1-2 pounds every week. Establishing a definite timeline when aiming to accomplish your objectives. Remember that intermittent fasting cannot be considered a quick fix that produces immediate results. It might require a few weeks or even months to witness noteworthy advancements.

Be practical regarding your fasting routine and the level of commitment you can afford. Steer clear of overexerting yourself or establishing impractical goals that could result in frustration or exhaustion. Bear in mind, the key to achieving success with intermittent fasting is by being unwaveringly committed and persevering.

Suppose your intention is to enhance your overall well-being by adopting intermittent fasting. One approach to consider is to establish a target of refraining from food for 16 hours each day and consuming all your daily meals within a restricted 8-hour timeframe. You could also establish a goal of reducing your sugar and processed food intake and increasing your consumption of fruits and vegetables.

Tips for Sticking to Your Plan

Sticking to an intermittent fasting plan can be challenging, especially if you're new to the concept. Here are some tips that can help you stay on track:

Start Slow

If you're just starting with intermittent fasting, it's crucial to proceed gradually and introduce it into your routine. Going from eating all day to not eating for an extended period can be difficult, both physically and mentally. Instead of jumping into a more aggressive fasting plan, start with a less restrictive plan like a 12:12 or 14:10 plan. The strategies entail refraining from food for either 12 or 14 hours per day and consuming meals only within a 12 or 10-hour timeframe, correspondingly. As you start feeling at ease with fasting, try extending the period without food little by little, adding an extra hour or two.

For example, when I first started intermittent fasting, I began with a 12:12 plan. My morning meal would be at 8 in the morning and I would conclude my final food intake at 8 in the evening. After some time, I extended my fasting period to 14 hours, and finally decided to adopt an 18:6 schedule, which involves fasting for 18 hours and eating meals during a 6-hour timeframe.

Stay Busy

One of the biggest challenges of intermittent fasting is resisting the temptation to break your fast. Being occupied can be beneficial in this scenario. Engaging in activities or tasks that keep you mentally or physically engaged during your fasting period can help take your mind off food and reduce the temptation to break your fast.

For example, during my fasting period, I would schedule a workout or a yoga class. I might strategize to make up for lost time by either completing pending tasks or indulging in some reading. These activities kept me engaged and helped me stay on track with my fasting plan.

Focus on Nutrient-Dense Foods

After completing your fast, it's crucial to prioritize the intake of nourishing foods that provide   your body with essential nutrients necessary for optimal functioning. Opting for nutrient-dense foods, which are rich in vitamins, minerals, and other essential nutrients, can help reduce cravings and prevent overeating during your eating window.

For example, I would break my fast with a green smoothie or a salad packed with vegetables and healthy fats like avocado or nuts. I would also include lean protein like grilled chicken or fish. These foods not only provided me with the nutrients my body needed but also helped me feel full and satisfied.

After careful consideration, incorporating intermittent fasting into your lifestyle can potentially bring about significant improvements in your overall well-being. However, it's essential to be careful and start slowly when trying out this nutritional routine. Starting with a less restrictive plan, staying busy, and focusing on nutrient-dense foods can help you stick to your fasting plan and achieve your health goals. Remember that personalized customization is important when it comes to intermittent fasting, and it should be based on your specific requirements and inclinations. Stay attuned to your body's signals and modify your fasting regimen as necessary.

Choosing the Right Fasting Plan

For women who are over 60, intermittent fasting can be a beneficial approach to preserving their overall health and happiness. However, selecting the appropriate strategy that aligns with their specific objectives and way of life is critical. Here are some suggestions with real-life examples for intermittent fasting plans that can work well for women over 60:

❖ Time-Restricted Eating: Time-restricted eating has become a trendy way of intermittent fasting. The method requires one to eat food within a designated timeframe and fast for the remaining hours of the day. Women aged over 60 may benefit from a 16:8 plan, which includes an 8-hour eating window and a 16-hour fasting period. This plan is adaptable and can be modified to fit personal schedules and inclinations.

Mary, a 65-year-old woman who was struggling with weight gain and high blood pressure, opted to give the 16:8 time-restricted eating strategy a shot, after seeking advice from her physician. Her new routine consisted of having meals solely from noon to 8 pm and abstaining from any food intake for the remainder of the day. She found that this plan was easy to follow, and within a few weeks, she noticed significant weight loss and a drop in her blood pressure.

❖ The 5:2 Fasting Plan: One way to manage weight and insulin sensitivity for women over 60 is the 5:2 fasting approach, which consists of maintaining a regular diet for five days of the week and reducing calorie intake to 500-600 calories for the other two days.

Linda, a 70-year-old woman who struggled with diabetes for many years, opted to give the 5:2 fasting regimen a try, following a discussion with her physician. For a couple of days every week, she ate only 500-600 calories and had a healthy, well-balanced diet for the rest of the week. She discovered that her glucose levels improved and that she could decrease the amount of medication she was taking.

❖ Alternate-Day Fasting: Every second day, alternate day fasting requires abstaining from food and consuming a typical diet on the remaining days. This plan can be more challenging, but it can be effective for women over 60 who want to lose weight or improve their metabolic health.

Susan, a 68-year-old woman who had been struggling with high cholesterol levels, chose to adopt a new eating pattern that involved alternating between days of fasting and eating a balanced diet. Within a few months, she noticed a significant drop in her cholesterol levels, and she felt more energetic and healthier overall.

As a general observation, women over the age of 60 can potentially benefit from intermittent fasting as a means of preserving their physical and mental health. However, it is highly recommended to seek the advice of a medical practitioner prior to initiating any new dietary or fasting regimen. Moreover, pay attention to your body's responses and adapt accordingly to prevent any adverse effects and maintain a positive state of well-being.

Starting Your Intermittent Fasting Plan

Consider the following useful pointers for designing your meals while intermittently fasting:

Nutrient-Rich Foods

To make the most of your diet, prioritize foods that are packed with essential nutrients that your body needs for optimal performance and energy levels. These foods include:

❖ Vegetables: Leafy greens, cruciferous vegetables, peppers, and mushrooms are all excellent sources of vitamins, minerals, and fiber.

❖ Fruits: Berries, apples, and citrus fruits are excellent choices because they are loaded with fiber and antioxidants.

❖ Whole grains: Brown rice, quinoa, and whole wheat are all healthy options rich in fiber and complex carbohydrates.

❖ Lean Proteins: A well-rounded diet could include protein from chicken, fish, eggs, or tofu to feel full and satisfied.

❖ Healthy fats from sources like nuts, seeds, avocado, and olive oil can also contribute to a feeling of fullness.

Hydration

Staying hydrated is essential during intermittent fasting. To prevent dehydration, make sure to drink enough non-caloric drinks such as water and herbal tea when fasting.

Portions

It's important to be mindful of the portions you eat to avoid overeating. Try using smaller plates and bowls to regulate the amount of food you eat, and stop eating once you feel full.

Meal Timing

When planning your meals, consider your daily schedule to ensure you have access to healthy options when you need them. If you anticipate a hectic schedule, it's wise to schedule a heartier breakfast to sustain your energy and concentration levels for the rest of the day.

Keep it Balanced

To maintain a healthy diet, eat meals that are well-rounded and consist of different food groups that can supply the essential nutrients and energy that your body needs. A properly balanced meal should contain a portion of low-fat protein, a portion of whole grain, and enough vegetables.

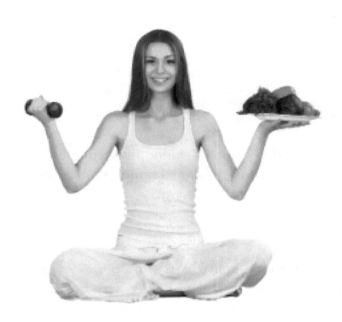

Conclusion: Healthy Lifestyle Habits

Living a healthy lifestyle shouldn't be overlooked. It's even more critical as we grow older and become more susceptible to chronic illnesses, such as heart disease, diabetes, and arthritis. A healthy lifestyle involves physical activity, rest, stress management, healthy eating, and community support to achieve overall well-being.

Staying active is one of the critical components of a healthy lifestyle. Engaging in physical exercise not only enhances the body's strength but also assists in mitigating the likelihood of long-term health issues, such as cardiovascular disease and stroke. Activities such as brisk walking, cycling, swimming, or strength training can be tailored to suit individual preferences and fitness levels. For example, my grandmother enjoys practicing yoga for flexibility and balance, which also helps to reduce her risk of falls.

Getting enough rest is crucial for the body to repair and rejuvenate. Getting sufficient and quality sleep is crucial in reducing the likelihood of developing chronic diseases, including diabetes and obesity. I personally experienced challenges with sleep deprivation, which affected my productivity and focus during the day. However, making changes to my sleep environment, such as following a regular sleep schedule and avoiding screen time before bed, has enhanced my sleep quality, leaving me feeling refreshed during the day.

Another crucial element of living a healthy lifestyle is effectively managing stress. Stress can have adverse effects on physical and mental well-being, causing conditions like anxiety, depression, and even chronic illnesses like heart disease and diabetes. By incorporating mindfulness practices such as meditation and deep breathing exercises, stress levels can be minimized, leading to an overall sense of well-being. Furthermore, engaging in relaxing hobbies such as gardening, reading, or painting can also assist in reducing stress.

In conclusion, living a healthy lifestyle is essential for general well-being, especially as we become older.

Suggestion list

❖ Spend a few hours of the day in someone's company or make a phone call to a loved one.

❖ Read, listen to music, draw, do a puzzle or gardening.

❖ Walk, exercise or do chair yoga if the weather is bad and you prefer to stay home.

❖ Help others and ask for help if you feel the need.

❖ Smile and laugh as frequently as possible.

❖ Don't focus on your diet but on your overall well-being.

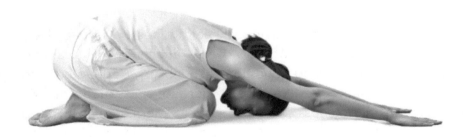

Book 2

Intermittent Fasting for Women Over 60

Your 28-day Intermittent Fasting 5/2 Plan

The 5/2 strategy calls for keeping a regular diet for five days while reducing caloric intake to 500–600 calories for two days that aren't consecutive.

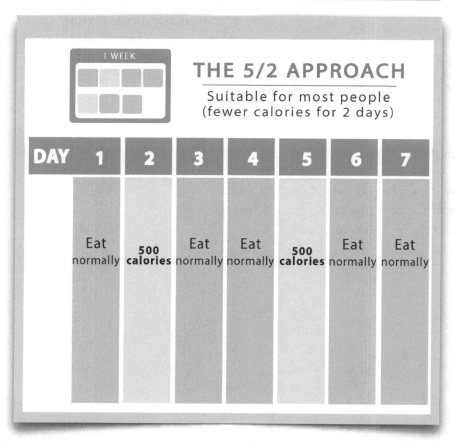

See here an example of guidelines for a 28-day meal plan during intermittent fasting.

Breakfast:

A bowl of creamy Greek yogurt mixed with fresh and tangy mixed berries sprinkled with crunchy chia seeds.

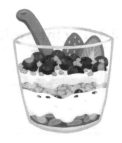

Midday meal:

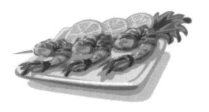

A colorful bowl of mixed greens, accompanied by savory and succulent grilled shrimp topped with slices of ripe avocado.

Evening meal:

A steaming bowl of hearty lentil soup, paired with a roasted sweet potato on the side.

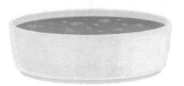

Day 2 (500-600 calories)

Breakfast:

Black coffee or herbal tea.

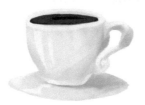

Midday meal:

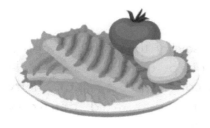

Char-grilled poultry chest, protein-rich quinoa, and oven-baked vegetables.

Evening meal (small portion):

Oven-cooked salmon, fiber-packed brown rice, and gently cooked broccoli.

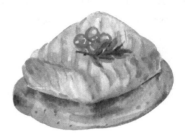

Day 3 (Eat normally)

Breakfast:

Fluffy eggs mixed with leafy spinach and earthy mushrooms.

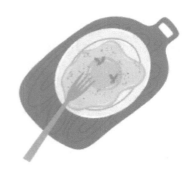

Midday meal:

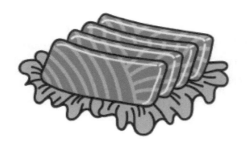

A savory tuna medley atop a crisp bed of lettuce accompanied by juicy cherry tomatoes and crunchy cucumbers.

Evening meal:

Tender beef slices tossed in a wok with a blend of colorful veggies, served over nutty brown rice.

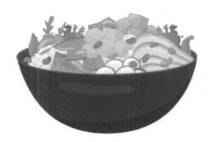

Breakfast:

Whole grain toasted bread garnished with slices of avocado and tomato.

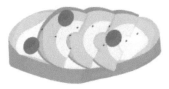

Midday meal: Mixed greens salad
with croutons and chicken, topped with Caesar dressing.

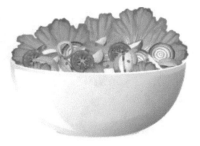

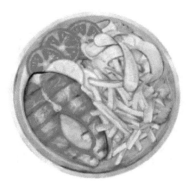

Evening meal:

Grilled salmon along with roasted asparagus and a side of sweet potato fries.

Breakfast:

Black coffee or herbal tea.

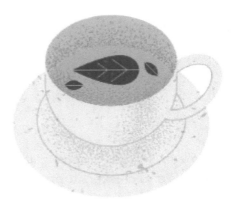

Midday meal: A hot bowl of tomato soup accompanied by a grilled cheese sandwich, toasted to perfection.

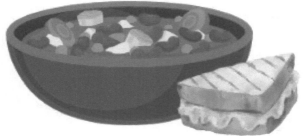

Evening meal (small portion):

Oven-baked juicy chicken thighs served with roasted Brussels sprouts and fluffy quinoa on the side.

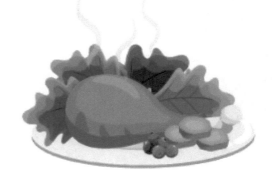

Breakfast:

Prepare a healthy green smoothie by blending kale, spinach, banana, and almond milk.

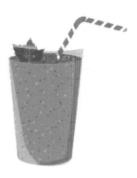

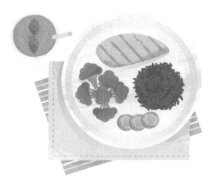

Midday meal:

Cook a juicy chicken breast on the grill and serve with a mix of leafy greens and quinoa.

Evening meal:

Whip up a delicious vegetable stir-fry by sautéing tofu and pairing it with brown rice.

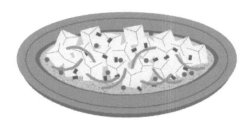

Breakfast:

A cup of milk and pancackes..

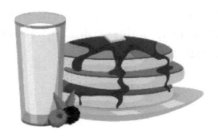

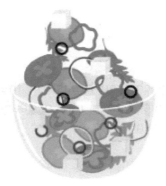

Midday meal: A medley of fresh greens, juicy tomatoes, salty feta cheese, briny olives, and tender grilled chicken.

Evening meal: A nutritious baked sweet potato filled with creamy black beans, buttery avocado, and zesty salsa.

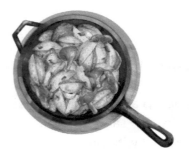

Day 8 (Eat normally)

Breakfast: A hot beverage made from black coffee beans, or a tea brewed from medicinal herbs.

Midday meal: A flame-grilled piece of lean chicken meat accompanied by an assortment of fresh leafy greens and oven-cooked veggies.

Evening meal: A fillet of salmon cooked in the oven and served with quinoa, a high-protein grain-like seed, and steamed broccoli.

Day 9 (500-600 calories)

Breakfast: Black coffee or herbal tea.

Snack: A combination of Greek yogurt, a medley of berries, and Chia seeds.

Midday meal: Grilled shrimp served with a mix of greens and avocado.

Evening meal (small portion): A warm bowl of lentil soup accompanied by roasted sweet potato on the side.

Day 10 (Eat normally)

Breakfast: Mashed eggs with spinach and mushrooms.

Midday meal: Tuna mix on top of a layer of lettuce with cherry tomatoes and cucumbers.

Evening meal: Stir-fried beef with diverse vegetables and whole-grain brown rice.

Day 11 (Eat normally)

Breakfast: Toast made from whole grains topped with avocado and tomato slices.

Midday meal: A salad made with mixed greens, croutons, and chicken seasoned with Caesar dressing.

Evening meal: Grilled salmon accompanied by roasted asparagus and sweet potato fries.

Day 12 (500-600 calories)

Breakfast: Black coffee or herbal tea.

Snack: Mix together rolled oats and almond milk in a jar, add sliced bananas and a sprinkle of cinnamon, then chill it overnight for a ready-to-eat breakfast or snack.

Midday meal: Warm up a homemade tomato soup and pair it with a grilled cheese sandwich that's been toasted to perfection.

Evening meal (small portion): Cook a delicious dinner of crispy chicken thighs in the oven, then serve them alongside roasted Brussels sprouts and fluffy quinoa.

Day 13 (Eat normally)

Breakfast: A blended drink made with green vegetables such as kale and spinach, a banana, and almond milk.

Midday meal: Grilled chicken breast with a mix of greens and quinoa.

Evening meal: Stir-fried vegetables with tofu and brown rice.

Day 14 (Eat normally)

Breakfast: Unsweetened coffee made from dark roasted beans, or a warm beverage made from steeped herbs. Oats prepared the night before mixed with almond milk, sliced banana, and a pinch of cinnamon.

Midday meal: A dish consisting of leafy greens, chopped vegetables, chunks of tangy feta cheese, flavorful olives, and grilled chicken pieces seasoned with herbs and spices.

Evening meal: A baked sweet potato served with a mixture of cooked black beans, diced creamy avocado, and a tangy tomato salsa made with fresh herbs and spices.

Day 15 (Eat normally)

Breakfast: Eggs mixed with spinach and mushrooms, cooked in a pan until scrambled.

Midday meal: A bowl filled with quinoa, grilled chicken, and roasted vegetables.

Evening meal: Salmon fillet grilled to perfection, accompanied by brown rice and steamed broccoli.

Day 16 (500-600 calories)

Breakfast: Black coffee or herbal tea.

Midday meal: Barbequed shrimp served with a combination of different types of green leaves and sliced avocado.

Evening meal (small portion): A bowl of lentil soup paired with a roasted sweet potato dish.

Day 17 (Eat normally)

Breakfast: Enjoy a serving of whole wheat bread topped with creamy mashed avocado and thinly sliced tomatoes.

Midday meal: Chicken Caesar salad made with a variety of greens and seasoned croutons.

Evening meal: Cook up some beef stir-fry with a mix of vegetables and serve it with brown rice.

Day 18 (Eat normally)

Breakfast: Combine oats with almond milk, banana, and cinnamon in a container, let it sit overnight for a nutritious breakfast.

Midday meal: Enjoy a warm bowl of tomato soup and pair it with a crispy grilled cheese sandwich on the side.

Evening meal: Bake chicken thighs until golden brown and juicy, then serve them with roasted Brussels sprouts and quinoa for a tasty and balanced dinner.

Day 19 (500-600 calories)

Breakfast: Black coffee or herbal tea.

Midday meal: Cook a chicken breast on the grill and serve it with a mixture of greens and quinoa.

Evening meal (small portion): Prepare a vegetable stir-fry consisting of tofu and brown rice.

Day 20 (Eat normally)

Breakfast: A serving of Greek yogurt combined with a medley of assorted berries and Chia seeds.

Midday meal: Greek greens with feta cheese, olives, and grilled poultry.

Evening meal: Cooked sweet potato with black legumes, avocado, and spicy sauce.

Day 21 (Eat normally)

Breakfast: Scrambled eggs combined with spinach and mushrooms.

Midday meal: A quinoa-based bowl served with grilled chicken and roasted vegetables.

Evening meal: A grilled salmon entree accompanied by brown rice and steamed broccoli.

Day 22 (Eat normally)

Breakfast: Blend Greek yogurt with Chia seeds and top it off with mixed berries for a nutritious breakfast.

Midday meal: Cook some grilled shrimp and serve it with a mix of greens and sliced avocado for a delicious lunch.

Evening meal: Make a wholesome lentil soup and serve it with a side of roasted sweet potato for a satisfying dinner.

Day 23 (500-600 calories)

Breakfast: Black coffee or herbal tea.

Midday meal: Salad made of chicken, mixed greens, and crispy bread cubes, with Caesar dressing.

Evening meal (small portion): Stir-fried beef strips, mixed vegetables, and steaming brown rice.

Day 24 (Eat normally)

Breakfast: Prepare a bowl of oats the night before by soaking them in almond milk, then add a sliced banana and sprinkle cinnamon on top.

Midday meal: Indulge in the comforting combination of a hot bowl of tomato soup and a grilled cheese sandwich to accompany it.

Evening meal: Bake some chicken thighs in the oven and serve them with roasted Brussels sprouts and quinoa as side dishes.

Day 25 (Eat normally)

Breakfast: Make a vibrant smoothie with kale, spinach, banana, and almond milk.

Midday meal: Cook chicken breast on the grill and serve with a mixture of greens and quinoa.

Evening meal: Stir-fry a variety of vegetables, tofu, and serve with brown rice.

Day 26 (500-600 calories)

Breakfast: Black coffee or herbal tea.

Midday meal: A mixture of vegetables such as lettuce, tomatoes, cucumbers, onions, and bell peppers with crumbled tangy white cheese made from sheep's milk, briny small pickled fruits, and char-grilled slices of tender poultry meat.

Evening meal (small portion): A root crop that is cooked by baking until tender and served with seasoned black legumes, slices of buttery green fruit with a creamy texture, and a condiment made from chopped onions, tomatoes, chili peppers, and lime juice.

Day 27 (Eat normally)

Breakfast: Whisked eggs combined with spinach and sliced mushrooms, cooked until fluffy and served hot.

Midday meal: A bowl of protein-rich quinoa mixed with grilled chicken and roasted veggies, for a variety of flavors and textures.

Evening meal: A juicy grilled salmon fillet served alongside a side of fluffy brown rice and steamed broccoli for a balanced and healthy dinner.

Day 28 (Eat normally)

Breakfast: Combine Chia seeds, mixed berries, and Greek yogurt for a healthy breakfast.

Midday meal: Enjoy a lunch of mixed greens and avocado paired with grilled shrimp.

Evening meal: Savor a warm and nourishing lentil soup with a side of roasted sweet potato for dinner.

WELL DONE!

Hungry? Here some snack ideas:

❖ Cut whole grain bread into slices and top with smashed avocado and sliced tomatoes.

❖ Combine low-fat fruit yogurt and let cool in the freezer for half an hour. Enjoy it like ice cream.

❖ Cut an apple into thin slices and sprinkle it with coconut flakes and cinnamon. Eat it along with a cup of herbal tea.

❖ Slice some carrots and celery and make a sauce with yogurt, garlic, salt and herbs. Use the sauce as a dressing.

Notes

❖ It's important to ensure that meals are balanced and contain a good mix of protein, healthy fats, and complex carbohydrates.

❖ To succeed with intermittent fasting, it's crucial to keep yourself well hydrated by drinking sufficient water during the day.

❖ While the provided plan can serve as a helpful reference point, it's equally important to pay attention to your body's signals and adjust your approach according to what works best for you as an individual.

Recipes
for
Intermittent Fasting

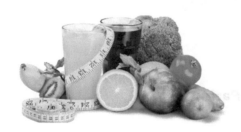

Breakfast Recipes

Overnight Oats

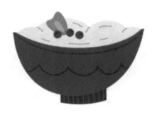

Mix together some rolled oats, almond milk, Chia seeds, vanilla extract, and sweetener of your choice in a mason jar. Keep it in the refrigerator overnight and garnish it with fresh berries and nuts the next morning.

Avocado Toast

Take a slice of whole-grain bread and heat it until toasted. Then, spread some mashed avocado on top of it, and sprinkle some chili flakes. Lastly, top it off with a poached egg.

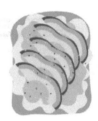

Greek Yogurt Parfait

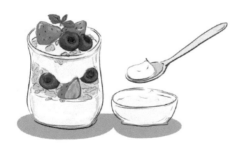

Arrange a delicious and healthy breakfast by layering some Greek yogurt, mixed berries, and granola in a jar. To make it sweeter, you may opt to put a dash of honey or maple syrup.

Egg and Veggie Scramble

Sauté diced bell peppers, onions, and spinach in a non-stick pan. Add in whisked eggs and cook until scrambled.

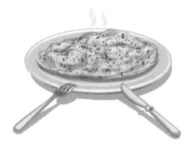

Chia seed pudding

A delicious breakfast option is Chia seed pudding, which is simple to make. Simply combine chia seeds with coconut milk and the sweetener of your choice. Let the mixture sit in the refrigerator overnight, and then add your favorite fresh fruit on top in the morning.

Lunch Recipes

Grilled Chicken Salad

Prepare a scrumptious salad featuring a perfectly grilled chicken breast, delicately sliced into thin pieces. Mix together some leafy greens, cherry tomatoes, and sliced cucumbers, then lightly coat with a vinaigrette dressing.

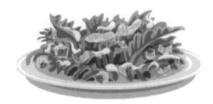

Lentil Soup

Prepare a dish of cooked lentils by combining them with diced vegetables such as carrots, onions, and celery in vegetable broth. Add seasoning in the form of cumin, turmeric, and coriander. Serve the meal while it's still steaming and include a piece of whole grain bread.

Cauliflower Fried Rice

Use a food processor to chop cauliflower until it resembles the texture of rice grains. Sauté with mixed vegetables like peas, carrots, and onions. Add in a scrambled egg for protein and season with soy sauce.

Tuna Salad Wrap

Combine canned tuna with finely chopped celery, red onion, and a spoonful of Greek yogurt. Wrap in a whole-grain tortilla with sliced avocado and arugula.

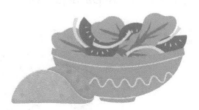

Chickpea and Vegetable Stew

Cook chickpeas with mixed vegetables like zucchini, squash, and tomatoes in vegetable broth. Season with paprika, cumin, and coriander. Serve hot with a side of brown rice.

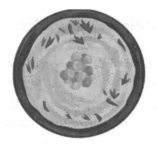

Dinner Recipes

Grilled salmon with roasted vegetables

Cook a piece of salmon and present it alongside some roasted veggies, like broccoli, asparagus, or zucchini.

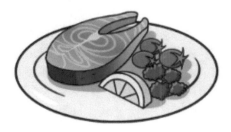

Turkey chili

Prepare a quantity of chili using minced turkey, legumes, diced tomatoes, and seasoning. Present the dish alongside a supplementary portion of either a salad or roasted vegetables.

Cauliflower fried rice

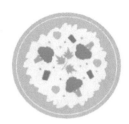

Make a healthier version of fried rice by using cauliflower rice instead of regular rice. Incorporate protein options like chicken or tofu and complement them with vegetables to create a healthy and nourishing dish.

Baked sweet potato with black beans and avocado

Prepare a delicious yam and add black beans, chopped avocado, and a scoop of Greek yogurt on it. This dish is rich in protein and healthy fats.

Grilled chicken with mixed greens

Grill a chicken breast and serve it on top of a bed of mixed greens. Add in some roasted vegetables or a side of quinoa for a well-rounded meal.

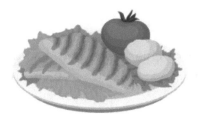

Dessert Recipes

As desserts are often high in sugar and calories, it can be challenging to find suitable options for intermittent fasting. Here are five dessert recipes that are delicious and easy to make while still being mindful of calorie intake:

Baked Apples with Cinnamon and Walnuts

Core and slice 2-3 apples, place in a baking dish.

Mix 1 tsp cinnamon with 1 tbsp honey and drizzle over apples.

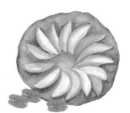

Scatter diced walnuts over the surface and bake in an oven preheated to 375°F for approximately 20-25 minutes.

Chia Seed Pudding

Blend together 1/4 cup of chia seeds and 1 cup of unsweetened almond milk, ensuring the milk is free from any additional sweetening agents.

Combine a teaspoon of vanilla extract with either one tablespoon of honey or one tablespoon of maple syrup.

Completely blend the components and put them in the fridge for at least two hours, or overnight.

Serve with fresh berries on top.

Chocolate and Almond Butter Cups

Melt half a cup of bittersweet chocolate with a double boiler or a microwave.

Cover the inside of a muffin tin with cupcake liners and add a bit of melted chocolate into every liner.

Place a teaspoon of almond butter in every cup, followed by pouring the rest of the melted chocolate on top.

Freeze for 20-30 minutes, and enjoy!

Berry and Fruit Yogurt Parfait

Place half a cup of plain Greek yogurt, half a cup of mixed berries, and a quarter cup of granola in a glass or jar, layering them one on top of the other.

If you like, you can gentle pour a bit of honey or maple syrup on top.

Peanut Butter and Banana "Ice Cream"

Freeze 2 ripe bananas, then blend in a food processor or blender until smooth and creamy.

Add 1-2 tbsp peanut butter and blend again.

Serve immediately or freeze for later.

Strategies for Staying Motivated

Here are three strategies to keep you motivated during an intermittent fasting plan:

Keep a Journal

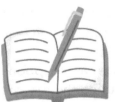

Keeping a journal or a diary can be a helpful strategy in monitoring your progress and maintaining your drive while going through a period of fasting. In your journal, you can write down your goals, track your fasting and eating patterns, and document how you feel each day.

By doing so, you can gain insights, identify patterns, and maintain a sense of accountability, ultimately enhancing your fasting journey.

For example, let's say you're trying to lose weight through intermittent fasting. By tracking your progress in a journal, you can see how much weight you've lost over time, how your body measurements have changed, and how your energy levels have improved. This powerful motivator can inspire and empower you to persevere in your fasting regimen and remain committed to your intended course of action.

Get a partner who will help you achieve your goals

Having someone responsible for keeping you accountable can serve as an effective method for reaching your objectives.

Find support from various avenues, such as a companion, a relative, or even an internet-based community. By checking in with each other regularly, you can provide support, motivation, and exchange tips and strategies for sticking to your plan.

For instance, if you're finding it challenging to resist temptation during your fasting period, your accountability partner can help you stay focused and motivated by reminding you of your goals. They can also offer encouragement and support when you're feeling discouraged or frustrated.

Focus on the Benefits

Focusing on the benefits of intermittent fasting can be a powerful motivator to stay committed to your plan. Several advantages are associated with it such as better weight control, elevated levels of vitality, and decreased inflammation.

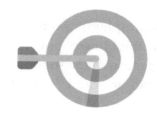

Moreover, there is evidence suggesting that intermittent fasting can lead to better cardiovascular health, enhanced cognitive performance, and increased lifespan.

Let's say you're struggling to maintain your fasting plan because you're feeling hungry and tired. By reminding yourself of the benefits, such as improved energy levels and weight loss, you can stay motivated to continue fasting. You can also remind yourself that the temporary discomfort is worth the long-term health benefits.

Tips for Overcoming Hunger

Here are three tips for overcoming hunger and food cravings during intermittent fasting:

Stay Hydrated

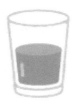

Staying hydrated has been covered several times in this book but it is necessary to reiterate because often people over 60 do not feel the need to drink and therefore forget to do so. Ensuring adequate hydration with water and other beverages that don't contain calories is essential while practicing intermittent fasting. When you fast, your body can lose a lot of water, leading to dehydration.

Adequate water intake eliminates dehydration and minimizes feeling hungry. Moreover, dehydration symptoms can be confused with hunger, so staying hydrated can assist in distinguishing between the two sensations.

To stay hydrated, carry a water bottle with you at all times. To make sure you stay hydrated all day long, use your phone to set up alerts reminding you to drink enough water. Additionally, you can mix it up by trying different types of non-caloric beverages, such as herbal teas.

Apart from drinking water, you can also increase your hydration level with fruits and vegetables that contain a significant amount of water, such as watermelon, strawberries, and cucumber. These edibles can increase satiety while you're fasting.

Practice Mindfulness

Practicing mindfulness exercises like taking deep breaths, meditating, or doing yoga can be effective in managing stress and anxiety levels, which in turn may decrease the likelihood of experiencing food cravings. These practices can also help you become more attuned to your body's hunger and satiety signals, serving as valuable tools for making informed decisions about meal timing and content.

To foster mindfulness, choose a calm environment where you can comfortably sit or recline. Take deep breaths, inhaling through your nose and exhaling through your mouth. Direct your attention to the physical experience of the air flowing in and out of your lungs as you breathe.

If you find it hard to stay focused on your breathing, you can try guided meditation apps like Headspace or Calm. Yoga is also a great way to practice mindfulness while getting some gentle exercise.

Distract Yourself

When you experience hunger pangs or cravings, it can be helpful to engage in a distracting activity to take your mind off food. Employing this technique can assist in resisting the temptation to eat and adhere to your fasting regimen.

Some great activities to distract yourself include going for a walk, talking to a friend, reading a book, or listening to music. You can also try more creative activities like painting, writing, or dancing. Explore a hobby that you find enjoyable and mentally stimulating. This could include activities such as playing a musical instrument, solving puzzles or crosswords, learning a new language, gardening, or even engaging in DIY projects. The key is to find something that piques your interest and challenges your cognitive abilities, providing you with a fulfilling and engaging pastime.

An alternative approach to keep your mind occupied is to prearrange your meals in advance. Doing so can keep you on track and driven while you are abstaining from food. Use a meal-scheduling app or document your meals in a personal logbook as a means of ensuring personal responsibility.

It's important to note that some level of hunger and cravings is normal during intermittent fasting, especially when you are first starting out. However, with time and practice, your body will become more accustomed to the fasting routine, and the feelings of hunger and cravings become less intense.

Conclusion: Importance of Nutrients

To provide the body with crucial nutrients and energy, it's important to consume a balanced diet consisting of whole foods. Eating a variety of different fruits, vegetables, lean sources of protein and healthy fats can help you keep a healthy body weight, support good digestion, and reduce the likelihood of developing long-term diseases. Personally, I enjoy cooking meals with fresh, seasonal ingredients, providing my body with all the essential nutrients it requires while also being fresh and delicious.

Lastly, additional resources such as community programs, support groups, and healthcare providers can help you live a healthy lifestyle and stay on track with wellness goals. Joining a walking group or fitness class can provide social support and accountability, while healthcare providers can offer guidance and resources for improving overall health.

From my personal experience, I have gained a lot by participating in a stress management support group. By interacting with individuals who had comparable encounters, I was able to develop valuable coping methods.

In conclusion, leading a healthy lifestyle is vital for overall well-being, particularly as we age. By integrating exercise, sufficient rest, stress coping mechanisms, nutritious food choices, and social support from our community, we can improve our overall health and lower the likelihood of developing long-term illnesses. Even minor, long-lasting alterations to our daily routines can enhance our well-being and help us accomplish our personal wellness objectives.

It's crucial to highlight that intermittent fasting is not a self-contained diet, but rather a specific pattern of eating. It should not be seen as a magical solution for losing weight or as a replacement for a well-balanced diet and healthy lifestyle. During eating periods, it's still important to consume nutritious foods and avoid overeating or binge eating.

Although intermittent fasting has shown promise in weight loss and enhancing health, it's not necessarily suitable for all individuals. Prior to embarking on an intermittent fasting routine, it's important to seek the advice of a medical expert to determine if it's safe and suitable for you and your health condition.

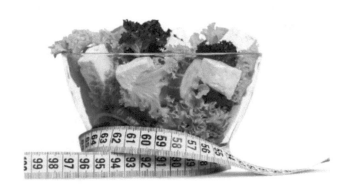

The Guided Intermittent Fasting Tracker

Keeping tabs on how you're doing with intermittent fasting can be a great way to stay motivated and focused on reaching your desired outcome. One potential benefit is the ability to recognize trends and modify your strategy to optimize your output. To make it easier for you to track your progress, we have developed a guided intermittent fasting tracker that you can use to monitor your fasting schedule, meals, and overall progress.

The tracker is designed to be user-friendly and simple to use, providing a clear overview of your fasting schedule and meals, as well as space to jot down notes and reflections. With this tool, you can easily track the duration of your fasts, the types of food you consume, and the impact that intermittent fasting is having on your health and well-being.

If you're just starting out with intermittent fasting or have already been doing it for a while, our customized monitoring tool can assist you in keeping up with your fasting routine and maximizing the benefits. With regular use, you can monitor your progress and adjust as needed, helping you achieve your goals and live a healthier, more balanced life.

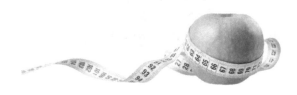

A Roadmap for Tracking and Measuring Results

Measuring your physical and mental characteristics is crucial to accurately track and assess the changes you will achieve from week to week. Physical changes are not the most important part of the process; your mind, clarity, energy, and the way you feel each day are also important elements to take into great consideration when evaluating the effectiveness of the diet. That is why I propose a roadmap that offers a model form for you to measure changes in your overall well-being, both before and after implementing the diet.

Start filling out the form by **measuring your body** on the first day of the diet and continue to measure yourself every week or every 15 days. Use a scale and tape measure to take the necessary measurements, following this template:

❖ Weigh yourself on a weighing scale

With the tape measure:

❖ Measure the circumference of your arms.

❖ Measure the circumference of your chest.

❖ Measure the circumference of your waist.

❖ Measure the circumference of your hips.

❖ Measure the circumference of your thighs.

Use the table below.

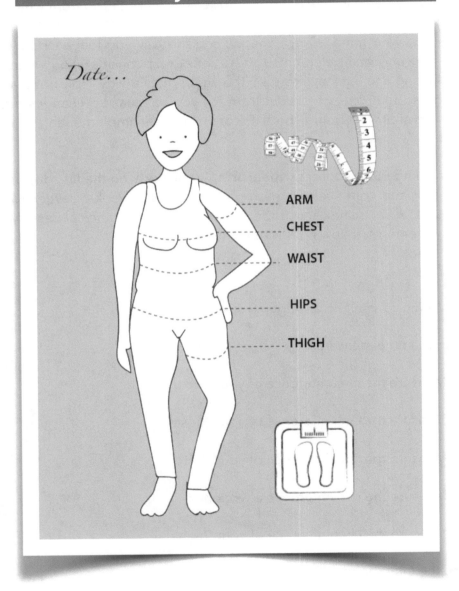

Date...

ARM

CHEST

WAIST

HIPS

THIGH

PHYSICAL

Date ....

	WEEK 1	WEEK 2	WEEK 3	WEEK 4
ARM				
CHEST				
WAIST				
HIPS				
THIGH				
WEIGHT				

NOTES

Intermittent Fasting - Emily William

Mental well-being

Continue filling out the form by measuring your **mental well-being.**

Give a score from 0 to 10 (where 0 corresponds to "dissatisfied" and 10 to "very satisfied") to each of these questions:

❖ Are you satisfied with your body?

❖ Are you energetic when you wake up in the morning?

❖ Do you feel strong?

❖ Do you feel confident about your ability to practice portion control?

❖ Are you able to distinguish mental hunger from physical hunger? (Clear Mind)

Use the table.

PSYCHOLOGICAL

Date

	M	T	W	T	F	S	S
HAPPY WITH YOUR BODY							
ENERGETIC							
STRONG							
CONFIDENT							
CLEAR MIND							

GIVE A SCORE FROM 0 TO 10 (WHERE 0 CORRESPONDS TO "DISSATISFIED" AND 10 TO "VERY SATISFIED")

NOTES

DAILY PLANNER

Date..........................

WEATHER

MOOD

WATER

TODAY'S AFFIRMATION

TOP 3 PRIORITIES

1 _____
_____

2 _____
_____

3 _____
_____

TO-DO LIST

☐ _____

☐ _____

☐ _____

☐ _____

☐ _____

☐ _____

☐ _____

☐ _____

DON'T FORGET

_____

_____

_____

BREAKFAST

1 _____
_____

2 _____
_____

3 _____
_____

LUNCH

1 _____
_____

2 _____
_____

3 _____
_____

DINNER

1 _____
_____

2 _____
_____

3 _____
_____

DAILY PLANNER

Date. . . . .

WEATHER ☀ ☁ ⛅ 🌧 ❄

TODAY'S AFFIRMATION

MOOD 😀 🙂 😐 🙁 😕 😞

WATER ⬡ ⬡ ⬡ ⬡ ⬡ ⬡

TOP 3 PRIORITIES

1 _____
_____
2 _____
_____
3 _____
_____

TO-DO LIST

☐ _____
☐ _____
☐ _____
☐ _____
☐ _____
☐ _____
☐ _____
☐ _____

DON'T FORGET

_____
_____
_____

BREAKFAST

1 _____
_____
2 _____
_____
3 _____
_____

LUNCH

1 _____
_____
2 _____
_____
3 _____
_____

DINNER

1 _____
_____
2 _____
_____
3 _____
_____

Day 3

DAILY PLANNER

Date.....................

WEATHER

MOOD

WATER

TODAY'S AFFIRMATION

TOP 3 PRIORITIES

1. _____
   _____
2. _____
   _____
3. _____
   _____

TO-DO LIST

- _____
- _____
- _____
- _____
- _____
- _____
- _____
- _____

DON'T FORGET

_____
_____
_____

BREAKFAST

1. _____
   _____
2. _____
   _____
3. _____
   _____

LUNCH

1. _____
   _____
2. _____
   _____
3. _____
   _____

DINNER

1. _____
   _____
2. _____
   _____
3. _____
   _____

DAILY PLANNER

Date......................

WEATHER ☀ ☁ ⛅ 🌧 ❄

TODAY'S AFFIRMATION

MOOD 😃 🙂 😐 😕 😔 😣

WATER ⬡ ⬡ ⬡ ⬡ ⬡ ⬡

TOP 3 PRIORITIES

1. _____
   _____
2. _____
   _____
3. _____
   _____

TO-DO LIST

☐ _____
☐ _____
☐ _____
☐ _____
☐ _____
☐ _____
☐ _____

DON'T FORGET

_____
_____
_____

BREAKFAST

1. _____
   _____
2. _____
   _____
3. _____
   _____

LUNCH

1. _____
   _____
2. _____
   _____
3. _____
   _____

DINNER

1. _____
   _____
2. _____
   _____
3. _____
   _____

Day 5

DAILY PLANNER

Date . . . .

WEATHER ☀ ☁ ⛅ 🌧 ❄

TODAY'S AFFIRMATION

MOOD 😄 🙂 😐 😕 😠 😢

WATER ◇ ◇ ◇ ◇ ◇ ◇

TOP 3 PRIORITIES

1 _____
_____

2 _____
_____

3 _____
_____

TO-DO LIST

☐ _____
☐ _____
☐ _____
☐ _____
☐ _____
☐ _____
☐ _____
☐ _____

DON'T FORGET

_____
_____
_____

BREAKFAST

1 _____
_____

2 _____
_____

3 _____
_____

LUNCH

1 _____
_____

2 _____
_____

3 _____
_____

DINNER

1 _____
_____

2 _____
_____

3 _____
_____

DAILY PLANNER

Date......................

WEATHER

MOOD

WATER

TOP 3 PRIORITIES

1. _____
2. _____
3. _____

TODAY'S AFFIRMATION

TO-DO LIST

- _____
- _____
- _____
- _____
- _____
- _____
- _____
- _____

DON'T FORGET

_____
_____
_____

BREAKFAST

1. _____
2. _____
3. _____

LUNCH

1. _____
2. _____
3. _____

DINNER

1. _____
2. _____
3. _____

DAILY PLANNER

Date........................

WEATHER

MOOD

WATER

TODAY'S AFFIRMATION

TOP 3 PRIORITIES

1 _____
_____
2 _____
_____
3 _____
_____

TO-DO LIST

☐ _____
☐ _____
☐ _____
☐ _____
☐ _____
☐ _____
☐ _____
☐ _____

DON'T FORGET

_____
_____
_____

BREAKFAST

1 _____
_____
2 _____
_____
3 _____
_____

LUNCH

1 _____
_____
2 _____
_____
3 _____
_____

DINNER

1 _____
_____
2 _____
_____
3 _____
_____

About the Author

Emily William is a renowned author and nutritionist specializing in intermittent fasting for women over 60. With over 20 years of experience in the health and wellness industry, Emily has dedicated her career to helping women achieve optimal health and wellness through healthy eating and lifestyle habits. She has authored several books, including the best-selling "Intermittent Fasting for Women Over 60," which provides practical tips and advice on how to safely and effectively incorporate intermittent fasting into a healthy lifestyle. Emily's expertise and passion for helping women achieve their health goals have made her a sought-after speaker and consultant in the industry. Her work has been featured in various health and wellness publications, and she continues to inspire and educate women around the world on the benefits of intermittent fasting for optimal health and wellness.

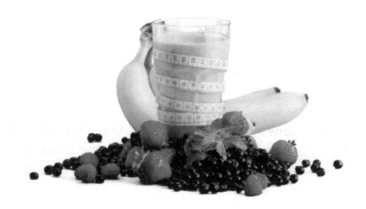

You can download the tables in printable format HERE

GET YOUR BONUS!

https://intermittentfasting.flyedition.com/

Your support means a lot to me and would be invaluable in spreading the word about my work. If you enjoy this book, please consider leaving a review!

Thank you

ISBN: 9798397027861

Made in United States
Troutdale, OR
05/28/2025

31713739R00060